MW01405283

THIS NOTEBOOK BELONGS TO

____

Made in United States
Orlando, FL
04 December 2021

11159665R00067